# Become & Stay Fit Forever

## The Holistic-Psychological Aspect of the Problem

Allyson Hodge

# Contents

# Introduction

It's after midnight, and you are getting out of bed, sneaking to the kitchen, and silently eating in front of the open refrigerator. Or, you are finally getting home after a long, tough day at work. All you want to do is sit on the couch in front of the TV and eat a whole carton of ice cream. Maybe you had a fight with your partner, or the children were screaming for hours. You think you may feel a bit better if you grab something tasty.

But after a while, you find yourself struggling to get into your clothes. It's time for diet and exercise. You know you can do it. You already succeeded the last time, and the time before, and even before. You could say you're an expert in getting back into shape. Wait, you can't. You have those ten extra kilos again. Sound familiar?

If you are one of those people who is always struggling with weight gain, counts every calorie, who has to work hard to lose some weight, just to put it back on again after a while, you are in the right place. In this book, we'll help you find the root of your problem, and solve it for good. So, when you finally get in shape again, you won't gain that extra weight back. We are going to break the cycle.

You will finally be free to rid yourself of all those plus-size pants and shapeless shirts, with no fear you may need them again.

Being caught in the cycle of gaining and losing weight is really frustrating. It can destroy your self-esteem, making you feel weak and powerless. We'll help you find out what's hidden in the background, and why you repeat the same process over and over again. Once you know what's the cause of it, you'll be able to face the right enemy.

## What's going on in your body

On the physical side, things seem pretty simple. The human body needs a certain amount of nutrients from food to function properly. It also requires enough movement to burn the energy it gets from food. When you eat the right amount of healthy, nutritious food, and move enough, your body is balanced. But, if you eat more food than your body actually needs, or do not burn enough calories through physical activity, that unused energy accumulates in your body as fat and makes you overweight. The calculation is simple, your body mass index (BMI) is the indicator of if you are overweight. It's a value derived from the weight and height of an individual. If your BMI is over 25, you are overweight. A BMI higher than 30 means a person is obese. If you have a problem with weight and want to lose some, what you need to do is to cut your calorie intake and boost energy burning. The healthiest way to do this is to develop a healthy diet low in calories and follow an exercise routine. This is not a secret, and it's nothing new for most of us. There are numerous weight loss diets, exercise programs, challenges, videos, books, coaches, and so on. It's up to you to try out different approaches and find out what works best for you. Some diets are based on choosing only specific kinds of food while avoiding others - from those which promotes eating only plants to those based on the belief that humans are carnivores exclusively, and many more in the middle of those two extremes. Some diet plans specify when you are allowed to eat. Then it's up to you to choose only the right, permitted foods, and have meals at the exact time of the day recommended. There are many more diets, plans, and approaches, and we would need a whole, separate book to cover that subject. Even then, it wouldn't be enough to describe all of them. That's why it's up to you to find the right system that makes you feel good. Whichever you choose, many people have succeeded in transforming their bodies using it. Every one of these diet programs has its good and bad sides, and each is efficient if you stick to it. And each is based on the same idea - cutting down your calorie intake.

The same thing applies to exercise. There are numerous programs and ways to burn calories. You can choose running, swimming, cardio, Pilates, Zumba dance, aerobics, and many more. You can work out at home, following instructions from YouTube, visit a gym every day, or hire a personal coach. The goal is the same - to burn as many calories as you can.

When you choose the right strategy and find the motivation, if you are committed and stick to your decisions, it's just a matter of time before you are going to succeed. It requires effort, it requires a lot of willpower and motivation, but in the end, it pays off. You see the progress and reach your goal.

And that should be all, right? You get fit and feel satisfied with your image in the mirror. If you learned how to live healthily, how to choose the right food, and work out regularly, you should never gain the weight again. But, it's happening. It's happening too often to be considered an accident. Everyone who went through this process of becoming fit, and then went back to their former state, has to ask why. Why is this happening? How is it possible, and why is that so common? May the problem lie somewhere else? What's attracting those extra kilos back? How can you get rid of them for good?

## What's hiding under the surface?

You can stay at the surface of the weight problem forever, trying every single pill for weight loss, and experiencing the yo-yo effect after every success. You'll have periods of temporary satisfaction, altering between periods of desperation about the extra weight as it comes back.

But how can you possibly not ask why it's happening? What is the real reason? You know that genetics has little to do with it. It's obvious overeating is the direct cause of the issue. But what's pushing you to eat more than you actually need? Yes, you are on the right track. There is always a reason inside you. It's hidden on a deeper level, and it's up to you to make an effort to find it and solve it. We are all different. That's why there's no one, universal psychological problem which is the same for all overweight people. But there are a few pretty common roots, typical scenarios that are common among those carrying extra weight. You will probably recognize yourself in some of them. We hope to help you find out what's the root of your impulse to eat more than you need and focus on the real cause of the problem, instead of focusing only on the symptoms. Being overweight is just a symptom of a deeper issue. That's why all the diets and exercise is only temporary. For lasting results, you need to pay attention to the main problem.

## Relationship with food

Like every other relationship in our lives, our relationship with food can be positive and joyful, but can also be dysfunctional. Why is that?

Like other important relationships, this one is built pretty early in our childhood. At the very beginning, it's a part of our relationship with the primary parent or guardian. As a baby is growing, these two relationships separate one from another. The first few years of life are the time when we form many connections. Food is associated with caring, comfort, peace, joy, and love. If all basic needs are met, and a child is fed and feels loved, he or she will build a healthy relationship with food. That means that, as an adult, the person will use food as fuel for the body, make healthy choices, and enjoy food, but not unhealthily. But, if any of a child's needs are not met, the chances are that this will impact his or her relationship with food later in life. How? You know those cases - a toddler is crying or having a meltdown, and a caregiver is offering food as a solution? "Oh, you are crying, that means that you are hungry!" If the child was thirsty, for example, after a few times he or she got food instead of a drink, what will they learn? When you are thirsty, have some food, and that may help. Or, maybe, the child was sad, nervous, angry, frustrated, or in a low mood, but still can't express those feelings in words, what is he or she learning? When you feel bad, get some food, and you'll feel better. Maybe it will only help for a moment, but that's how adults solve their bad moods.

In cases when a child has experienced a loss, trauma, or abuse, that will reflect on their relationship with food, too. The child you used to be becomes your inner child when you grow up. If the inner child is hurt, you'll always want to protect and comfort them. But if you are not aware of the cause, the ways you are trying to provide comfort may be more destructive than productive for you.

It is never too late to build a happy and healthy relationship with food. But first, you need to be aware of your patterns and habits and replace them with new, better ones.

Food is not here to make you happy. Food is not here to give you company. Not even to cure your boredom. It's here to fuel your body with nutrients and supply it with energy — nothing more, nothing less. Every other component you notice in your relationship with food means that you are trying to use it for something it wasn't created for.

## Thermostat

Have you ever noticed that you have a specific weight which seems to suit you the best? Everybody has it. If you eat as much as you want, not taking care of what you choose, how much weight would you gain? For one person it may be 68 kg, 82kg for someone else, 123kg for another. It's unique to each of us. What's your number? And why that one? Why not a few kilos more or less? It seems that we have some kind of inner thermostat which regulates our weight. That depends on many factors, on our beliefs about normal, low and high weight, our image of ourselves and the image of the perfect self. Although it's pretty stable, the good news is that you can take control over your weight thermostat and set it to your ideal weight. But that requires some effort to understand yourself and some work on self-development.

## Emotional eating

You are probably asking what food has to do with emotions. Well, it shouldn't have anything to do with them, but it does.

Comforting ourselves with food, binge eating, becoming addicted to certain foods - these are just a few kinds of emotional eating.

From our first day on the planet, we learn to connect food with love, warmth, acceptance, and comfort. And this is perfectly reasonable when you are a baby. Without love, a baby who depends on adults wouldn't survive. However, this connection between food and satisfaction is present even when you are grown up. As kids, we go through different phases, but adults still show us love and care through feeding us, and making food for us too. From early childhood, we learn to enjoy sweet tastes, and that association may comfort us even as adults.

There are many examples of emotional eating. In fact, every time you eat without feeling hungry is a kind of emotional eating. There's always some emotion in the background of this behavior. You may eat because you feel weak and experience a drop in sugar levels. But, if you dive deeper, you'll perhaps find out that you are feeling stressed. Stress drains your energy, your brain is using more sugar than it should, and that's the same process as if you had many apps open on your phone, working in the background. Stress drains your batteries. And the cause of stress is psychological.

Even without those sugar level drops, you may eat every time you feel stressed. The reason is obvious - you want to distract yourself from an unpleasant event or thoughts, and to feel better immediately - even just for a moment. Maybe you subconsciously believe that food will give you extra power to deal with the problem.

Many of us have an eating impulse without a real hunger trigger when we are worried, anxious, nervous, or feeling blue. The thought in the background is pretty much this, "Maybe I can't do anything about this, but there is always something I can do to feel better – eat!"

The same "cure" is often used for boredom. When you are bored, uninspired or lack motivation, it would be much more constructive to find a productive activity than to eat empty calories.

Many types of research have shown that people eat more when they lack sleep. When you are tired, you tend to crave energy from another source. That's the main reason for eating a chocolate bar to energize yourself quickly.

## Comfort food

Comfort food is food that has emotional value for someone. It may be nostalgic or sentimental, something that brings you back to your childhood or recalls happy memories. It's often high in calories, carbohydrates, or may require specific preparation. Different cultures all around the world have different typical comfort foods. It may also be specific for an individual.

Comfort food wouldn't be a bad thing if people didn't fall back on it so easily. This food is usually unhealthy. It's rich in calories, fat, salt, or sugar - foods such as ice cream, French fries, or chocolate, and it triggers our brain's reward system. That produces pleasure, and we temporarily feel better. As food has its purpose, using it for treating a bad mood has side effects. Comforting yourself with food to reduce stress is maladaptive behavior, responsible for bad eating habits and the obesity epidemic.

What is your favorite comfort food? Do you often treat yourself using this method? Next time you feel the need to get pampered and spoiled, try out some other way of doing so. Going to a spa, having a massage, lighting up scented candles, listening to music, or taking a walk may be a much better choice.

# Food addiction

Does it really exist?

Yes, it's real. Some kinds of food are addictive. There are some kinds of food and drink that we consume daily with no thought about its nutritional value. These are usually high-fat, salty and sweet foods or beverages. Consuming them causes a chemical reaction in the brain responsible for pleasure. Our brain produces the feel-good chemical - dopamine. That's why people can become addicted to the feeling linked to consuming unhealthy food.

We get reward signals which can be so strong that we don't notice natural signs of fullness. This leads to overeating, bad habits, and obesity.

So, a food by itself is not addictive, but you can easily become addicted to the good feeling it provokes.

# Switching

When it's about bad eating habits, we can talk about switching in any case when one eats food instead of addressing his or her real needs.

For example, it may be that you don't recognize thirst every time you feel it. You may believe it's hunger and eat instead of drinking water. That's not surprising considering that, from early childhood, people care more about feeding children than about hydrating them. That's why we often have no problem recognizing when we are hungry but skip drinking.

Hydrating sufficiently is a habit that we need to develop for a balanced, healthy lifestyle. Drinking water hydrates our cells and makes us feel energized and fresh while flushing out the toxins from our body. Taking in enough liquids will help you learn to recognize your needs, hydrate your body, and, besides that, you won't consume unneeded calories instead of it. So, next time you are going to get a snack, usually sweet, stop for a moment and ask yourself if maybe a glass of water is what you really need.

One more type of switching is what's going on when you lack sleep and eat instead. Sleeping is as crucial for our wellbeing as food, maybe even more. A human can go up to three days healthily without food, but hardly any time without sleeping. It's essential for our mind and body, and an irreplaceable way of charging, refreshing, and restoring ourselves. Sleeping is the time when your body and mind rest, gaining new energy and fixing little issues made during the day. When we lack sleep, we can't perform at our best. That's why we crave more food than we usually need. The chances are that the food we crave is sweet, because we need an immediate load of energy. An additional reason to this may be that our society fuels obesity by considering it perfectly normal to snack and eat more than required while underestimating the importance of rest and sleep. For example, it's nothing unusual to have pause to eat a sandwich or a bar of chocolate, but if you said you're going to sleep a little in the middle of a workday, that would hardly be well accepted.

Anyway, it's up to you to afford yourself enough rest during the day. An average adult needs six to eight hours of uninterrupted sleep, but that number varies from one person to another, and you need to find what works best for you. It depends on your age, gender, daily activity, and energy you need to perform at your best. It's good to be aware of being tired and prevent yourself from eating to cover for the lack of rest. When you go to the refrigerator between regular meals, consider going to bed instead. If you need rest, that's the only thing that will really help you. Eating food instead will supply you with a little energy, but many more calories.

Now, pay extra attention. This is the crucial point. Maybe you weren't aware of it. Perhaps you will be hearing it for the first time. And maybe it will change your life. It will give you a deeper insight and help you stay permanently fit. Ready?

Here's that most important type of switch:

## What you are trying to find in food is your inner peace.

Read that again. Read it as many times as you wish until you find that truth in yourself. Whatever your problem is, be it boredom or sadness, lack of self-esteem, or feeling powerless, what you are looking for is inner peace.

Finding it is the universal answer for any kind of emotional eating. It may sound a bit silly at first; you won't consciously looking for inner peace in food. But, if you think more about - when you are mentally in a good space, you don't feel all those poor emotions that make you seek reward. You don't suffer from a lack of joy, sadness, anger, resentment, or guilt. You don't think you are worthless or powerless. You don't depend on others to reassure you and approve of you. You don't need to seek comfort in the wrong places. Then you are able to heal all of your relationships, including your relationship with food.

So, although it may seem like a physical problem exclusively, obesity is actually a symptom of an emotional state, and a lack of inner peace.

That's the reason why lost weight so often happens to come back. If you do nothing about your mental space, no diet can give you permanent results. There really is something that attracts surplus weight like magic - it's your mindset. If you don't do something to change it and make it serve you, every struggle with undesired weight is hopeless. And it will stay this way forever - a battle. A healthy diet and exercise are great, and it must bring a result. But the only way to maintain that result permanently is to combine them with one more kind of diet - a mental diet.

Being on a mental diet is not as much a diet as a lifestyle. That means that you avoid negative thinking, work on changing your mindset, become more mindful, and work actively on finding your inner peace. That is the third crucial part in combatting a problem with weight or obesity. That is the part which is often missing, and the one we need to stay fit forever.

# How to help yourself

Whether you are religious or not, think about this idea - that Heaven and Hell exist. Both are in your head. You can mentally be in one or the other. It depends on your choices - your thoughts and emotions.

Here we will talk about what you can do to find that place of peace and happiness inside yourself. Some self-development techniques can help you. Practicing them, accompanied with a healthy lifestyle, is the key to becoming the best version of yourself. As we are not only one-dimensional beings, we are our soul, our mind and our body, all together and at the same time, you can't neglect your body and expect to be perfectly happy. Also, you can't focus only on something material, such as your body, food, taking calories in and burning them, exercise etc. - and expect lasting change. Your approach needs to be holistic, concentrating on your physical, mental and spiritual wellbeing. Only together, those three can bring you the life you deserve, full of joy.

# Introspection

## Address the real problem

The first step is to find out what's bothering you from the inside. As always, when we need to dive deep into our being, we'll begin from the surface. For the beginning, you need to do self-monitoring.

Don't try to change anything yet. Only focus on watching and noticing. Carefully look at your daily routine and eating habits and try to discern as many details as you can. What are you eating? When do you usually eat? In what environment do you have your meals? How often do you eat? Do you have snacks? When does that usually happen? What situations and circumstances trigger your impulse to eat? For example, you may regularly eat late at night, or like to eat a lot of candy when you feel stressed. Write down everything you notice that may be important to bring you insight about your eating, besides those when you are hungry.

Every time you feel the urge to eat something, stop for a moment, and ask yourself if it's really hunger that you are feeling. Is there any other emotion? Write down how you feel; that will help you to reveal your patterns and typical situations when you use food to solve something.

These notes will show you if you are overeating, eat too often, make unhealthy choices, and what circumstances trigger this behavior. You may notice that you are eating food to get some extra energy or comfort in specific situations - after a long, tough day, or after a fight or any other unpleasant event. Maybe you feel exhausted when the children are screaming, or you have an endless to-do list waiting. Or it's usually when you are expecting something stressful, such as an exam, a meeting or a presentation. Now you have an idea about what to pay attention to.

One more thing you may happen to notice - do you usually eat while watching television? Or are you typically having snacks while working on the computer? These links are not rare at all. But in this process, you will need to work on breaking them, too.

Before we go on with monitoring ourselves and tracking our eating habits, let's take a moment to talk about food connections.

If you are one of those people who is always snacking while watching TV, for example, try to be mindful about this. Decide to eat only at the dining table. Try to eat before sitting in front of the TV, without any snacks around. If you don't like this, which is not hard to understand when you are breaking a habit, you may try not to watch TV at all for some time. If this is too hard an option for you, try with tea or some other sugar-free drink. After a few days, you'll begin to enjoy a new, healthier habit - drinking tea while watching TV. That is a small, but powerful, change. Besides a lower-calorie intake, this will bring you back the feeling of power, of being in control of your life. If you can stop snacking while watching TV, you can make many other changes, too.

## Track your emotions

As we already said, emotions are the underlying cause of inadequate eating. So, the most important thing to pay attention to is tracking them. That will help you come to valuable insight and understand the complete picture. Once you know when you are doing what you want to stop and why are you doing it, you'll be able to prevent it and find better solutions instead.

Focus on your feelings during the day, especially in those moments when you want to chow down on something, or you crave a particular food. You can do this at the same time while paying attention to the circumstances. Include tracking your emotions into your self-monitoring process. When you write down the events and things that make you turn to food, stop for an extra moment, and ask yourself how you are. What do you feel? It is probably some unpleasant emotion. Is it fear? Anger? Are you stressed, nervous, anxious? Be honest with yourself. Being unaware of your feelings or separated from them will bring you nothing useful. It always turns into different psychological problems which cause physical symptoms, too. Be wise and make your problem with your weight work for you. How? Let it be your entrance into getting to know yourself better, becoming more mindful and improving your life. Treat it as a symptom of neglected emotions. Pay attention to what your soul is whispering. Perhaps it is screaming for your attention, and you are trying to shut it up by eating. It's not your stomach that is screaming; it's your soul. And it doesn't need more calories; it requires some soul food.

The first step in healing your soul is finding out what's not in balance below the surface. Recognize your emotions. Accept them, whether you like it or not. If you are scared, find out what is frightening you. Be clear with yourself, and then you will find more efficient cures than putting your emotions on hold while you snack on something. Don't ignore them anymore. If you are angry, understand why you are. Who has hurt you? Why are you suffering? Do you feel guilty? Why? What couldn't you forgive yourself for? Are you sad? Are you lonely? It would be better healing if you sit beside that refrigerator and cry all the tears out, rather than opening it to snack again. Don't be ashamed. It is human to have feelings. You can write about them if that would help you to get closer to them. Consider starting an introspection diary, where you can track your emotions. That will offer you a clear insight on which feelings make you think you are hungry.

## Are you trying to eat a problem?

We don't say you have such silly ideas. Perhaps you have never heard about this approach. But, there is a chance that you are, subconsciously, trying to move the problem out of your way. You want to make it disappear. "I can't do anything about this. I can't solve it," your mind thinks. "I want it to disappear. I will destroy it. I can eat the problem!" Your subconscious has a solution. It makes you eat compulsively without a hunger trigger, and without even thinking about why, what, and how much you are eating. Your autopilot does all of that, while you are not even consciously involved. These "solutions," of course, never work. By "eating your problem" you actually make it worse, because you don't pay real attention. You are ignoring the problem. Food never solved any problem except hunger, because it is not here to solve anything else. And, as you already know, a problem can't be eaten, except if your problem is a chocolate cake.

## What are you feeding?

By ignoring a real problem that's bothering you, you are making it worse. You are feeding it. The extra energy you get through food to cover it, hide it, or try to eat it, only makes your problem stronger. For example, if you are sad and eat to solve that emotion instead of facing it, you'll only become more miserable. You'll still have your initial sadness, plus you'll be sorry for eating all those unnecessary calories, you'll feel powerless because you couldn't resist a temptation, and hopeless because you anticipate you won't be able to change this behavior. You'll be miserable in your own eyes because of eating out of sadness, and then you'll have an impulse to eat even more because of that misery. That's a magic circle, and that's how things go from bad to worse.

## Are you trying to build up a wall to hide and protect yourself?

Eating more food than your body needs to perform well will make you overweight and undesirable. You know that. And you want to be fit and pretty. Or don't you? What a stupid question, you think, everybody wants to be desirable.

Well, not everybody. There are cases when one, subconsciously again, wants to be unnoticeable. The reasons can be different. You may have a jealous partner and want to avoid trouble by making yourself less attractive. Also, you may be keeping yourself from leaving a current relationship or marriage.

Or, more often, people who went through sexual abuse in childhood, are scared to be noticed or liked. They tend to cover their body with fat, to be as undesirable as they can.

Maybe you are too shy and want to hide behind a wall. Because there is no wall, you are building it.

You may also be building this "fat castle" to protect yourself from the world that you believe is a dangerous, scary place. If you live with a deep, fundamental fear from life, and are generally anxious, chances are this is the case. You are doing two things at the same time - comforting with food and hiding inside your overweight body.

## Are you incorrectly addressing your needs? What do you really need instead of food? What are you hungry for? How can you get it?

- Before anything else, are you rested? How did you sleep? Was it enough for you? Maybe you need to rest, to take a nap.

- Are you thirsty? Try your best to drink at least eight glasses of water per day. Not beverages like juice, soda, coffee, alcohol - just pure water. Remember to check this before you drink anything.

- How do you feel? Do you feel a lack of something? What is currently missing in your life? Do you lack love or approval? Maybe you would like a big hug, but there's no one beside you.

Address your needs correctly. Then you will know what constructively to do about it - to cry the pain out, to forgive, to visit a therapist, to talk to a friend.

If you are lonely, you should put some socialization into your schedule.

If you are bored, there are plenty of activities to solve that. Life is magical and full of colors, full of joy and excitement. You don't need to seek it in taste. Food can't entertain you. Food is not fun; it's only fuel for fun.

Think about the ways to get what you need. You can make a change. You can find what you are looking for. Giving up on everything you truly need and looking for comfort in food is a sign that you feel powerless. But power is still within you. Use it to break the cycle. Stop with the wrong choices and prepare your mindset to be your friend.

## Change your goals

As a society, we are used to fighting with weight, counting calories, beating ourselves up for our mistakes and imperfections, and chasing a certain number on the scale.

But who taught you that specific number would bring you happiness? What if the process is actually the reverse? What if you need to go in the opposite direction - to become happy, and then you can become fit? We are used to starting from the surface, but most often that's where we stay. What if you need to begin from the inside, with a lot of inner work?

'Till now, you know that is true. That is the way things actually go.

What about your goals?

Do you have them? We're thinking a specific goal, like losing 20 kg by April 29? No? If you have it, great. That means you already know about right goal settings. If not, that's not a problem.

We'll explain the basics about goal settings, and then see why it doesn't work here.

You need to have goals, big ones, and little ones to lead you in the right direction. Write them down, because that increases your chances to achieve them. A goal should be SMART:

Specific, for example - I want to pass the math exam.

Measurable - like I want to lose 15 kg.

Achievable and Realistic- I want to fly to the moon won't motivate anyone to take an action.

Time-Framed - One day, later, during my lifetime and so on are not deadlines. These words mean that you will achieve it probably never. You need to set the time for your goals - until next Sunday, this year, until November 16, and so on.

Now, you have set your goals. When it's about losing weight, most often, our goals sound like this: I want to lose 20 kg before (date).

And it is probably correctly set - it's specific, measurable, time-framed, and most often realistic and achievable. You set smaller goals, too. Most often they are to exercise x times a week, to stick to your eating plan, drinking enough water, and so on. And that's ok, too.

What's wrong then?

Two things.

First, we most often behave like we are punishing ourselves with strict and rigorous restrictions and not proper exercise. We beat ourselves up for every mistake, we are angry and disappointed if we don't strictly hold to this unnatural program. It's overwhelming. It's both physically and psychologically exhausting.

And here we come to another, a bigger problem, with these goals. No one would want to live like this forever. These programs, involving starving and hard exercise, are strictly time-framed, which helps us to hold on 'till the end. It's like penal servitude. When we finish it, it's over, and we can celebrate. We finally achieved the desired number on the scale, that's it! Besides, it's not. These programs do nothing about your mind, your mental attitude. That's why most of us go back to old habits. We haven't built new, healthier habits, or changed our approach. We've just served what we had to, and the change in kilos is only temporary. That's why it doesn't work.

If you want permanent change, it must begin from the inside. You need to rewire your mind and reprogram it.

And you obviously need to change the goals.

How?

Your weight goal doesn't need to just be smart. It should be even smarter.

Your goal shouldn't be to be skinny, but to be healthy. It shouldn't be temporary, but forever. Not like, "I'll try this new diet and work-out plan for the next two months." It should be more like, "I'll commit myself to becoming healthy. I exercise three times a week for the rest of my life. I'm not dieting; I eat healthily."

Don't set strict limitations, don't restrict food. That will only make you strive for forbidden food and feel like a failure.

What you need to set as a goal is to become the healthiest version of yourself, to have a strong, fully functioning body (and mind), while being kind and loving to yourself, and stay permanently healthy and fit.

Maybe it's not as specific and measurable as it is to chase that certain number on the scale, and "forever" doesn't sound like time-framed. However, if you change your approach, stop looking at weight loss as a particular project, and achieving the desired weight as part, but develop a healthy lifestyle instead, that will make it possible for you to keep the body permanently fit.

So, you won't be dieting anymore - you will choose healthy foods, the best for you.

You won't exhaust yourself with working out - you will enjoy the movement in honor of your body.

You won't struggle with weight - you will enjoy the full potential of your body.

# Change your beliefs

What do you believe about food, weight loss, yourself and your body? This is all very important because it determines your weight.

Commit some time to introspection again. This time you are looking for your limiting beliefs about these three things. What you need to dig up are all those things you learned during life, for example: "Food is bad, it's making me fat."

"It's easy to gain weight, but it's hard to lose it."

"Everybody gains weight with the years."

"That's my constitution and genetics; I'm destined to be chubby." "It's hard for me to lose weight."

"My body is ugly."

"I'm not good enough," and so on. Be patient, give yourself enough time to come to all those beliefs hidden under the surface that may make it hard for you to love yourself and your body, to have a healthy relationship with food, and achieving your healthy weight.

Once you dig them up into the daylight, it's time to change them into positive, supportive beliefs. How can you do that? Use affirmations.

For those who are not familiar with affirmations, these are affirmative sentences that we repeat as long as they're needed to become our new beliefs.

Beliefs are just thoughts that we have heard or said enough times to start believing in them. So, we will reverse the process, and start believing in the opposite. Always write your affirmations in a positive, confirmative tone, in the present.

For example:

"Food is good; it's fuel for my body."

"I choose healthy food."

"It's easy for me to eat healthily and move enough."

"My body is a wonderful miracle."

"I have a healthy, fully-functioning body."

"I love my body."

"I'm worth love."

"I love myself," and so on, in the same manner, until you change all the limiting beliefs with new, supportive ones.

Don't worry if your affirmations sound weird at the beginning. They are talking to your subconscious.

But, it's also essential that you take them as truth, not as lies to yourself. If an affirmation sounds like a lie, change it to believe it. For example, if you know you are overweight, it may seem insincere if you are saying, "I'm fit and healthy." It would be better for you to choose a more general option like, "I'm ready to become fit and healthy."

The right beliefs will support your weight-loss journey and enable you to rewire your mind and adopt the right mindset to stay fit forever.

# Visualization

Your subconscious doesn't make a difference between what's happening for real and what's just your imagination. That's why visualization is so powerful in creating reality. What you want to reach by visualizing is the feeling. Daydreaming helps you to feel the same emotions as you would if it was happening for real. By The Law of Attraction, your emotions are crucial in creating reality, so you will attract what you are visualizing.

Whether you believe in The Law of Attraction and creating reality or not, this technique will help you in reaching your desired weight and staying in good shape.

You can practice it as a part of meditation, after relaxing your whole body. Imagine yourself fit, healthy, and smiled. Imagine how do you feel in your perfectly-toned body. Enjoy the feeling and try to remember it. It's more powerful motivation than any motivational talk you may hear.

While drinking water, imagine how it takes away all the negativity from your body, all the extra calories you don't need and how it washes out all the toxins from your body.

You can also visualize a white light that is covering the whole body, bathing it, healing, and taking all the extra weight away. Your body becomes light and easy.

## Meditation

How can sitting and not burning calories help me lose weight?!

It really is strange if you focus only on the traditional approach that only counts calories and overlooks inner work.

But the truth is that our body is a reflection of what's going on inside our minds.

We need to understand why the problem with weight is happening, where we are making mistakes, why we can't maintain the results, and much more. That requires a lot of inner work. You need to question your thoughts and beliefs, confront your feelings, dig up past trauma and emotional triggers. All your negative experiences may have accumulated and manifested into an unhealthy weight.

Sitting still, in silence, relaxed, in a welcome state, allows you to ask yourself questions and come to the truth. You may get brilliant insight into why you are doing what you are doing, why you grab fast food or skip workouts. You can re-explore your motivations for weight loss and why you are sabotaging yourself. You can also become aware of some habits from your childhood, for example being told that you have to eat everything on your plate. All of these will help you to mentally prepare to stick to a weight loss regime, get and maintain your ideal weight. You will dig up your subconscious blocks, fears, and patterns that are standing in your way.

Finally, practicing meditation, you will find your inner peace, peace with food and your body. You will get a lot of improvement in your relationship with the most important person in the world - yourself.

Besides all that, meditation has an indirect impact on weight loss - it improves health overall, reducing stress, improving sleep, and rewiring the parts of the brain responsible for emotions that cause emotional overeating.

How to start?

Dedicate some time in a day (it may be as little as five minutes at the beginning) to spend in quiet, alone. Sit still or lie down and focus only on your breath. When you notice any thoughts popping up, just let it go and keep concentrating on your breathing. That's all. The goal is to relax the whole body and pay full attention only to your breath and becoming entirely present in the moment. By practicing, your focus will improve, and you will learn how to shut your mind off for some time.

Once meditation becomes part of your routine, and the personal exploration begins, you can apply this new awareness to other parts of your life, too. Meditation and mindfulness help us discover and overcome mental barriers we often make subconsciously.

## Mindfulness

What does it mean to be mindful?

That's being absolutely and consciously present in the moment with your whole being. That's our natural state, but we forgot it because of the modern life we live. Our minds too often jump into the past or the future, overlooking the only reality we have for real - the here and now. Becoming mindful (again) is a technique which can be learned and practiced. Learning to concentrate on the moment, noticing everything around you with all your senses, you will become more present. You'll become more aware of the world around you, yourself, and your body.

What does it have to do with weight loss?

Practicing mindfulness during the day, especially while you are preparing food, eating, or moving, will help you become aware of your unhealthy habits, choices, and triggers that work against your goals.

Mindful eating can get you a long way in your healthy journey. How to eat mindfully?

While preparing meals and eating, be present and focused on food. Try to notice as much as you can - the taste, the texture, the smells. Think about your food - how it's grown, how it's prepared. Eat only if you are in a good mood and your thoughts are positive. If you have some negative thoughts about the food you are eating, if you are suspicious about its quality or the way it's made, don't eat it. It's more harmful than good because you are not bringing in only materialized food, but also its energy.

Slow down, give yourself time to set your vibration, to become present and mindful while eating. Don't just gulp the food without thinking. Reconnect your mouth with your mind and pay attention to each bite with all of your senses.

Take time to be grateful for the food that gave its life to feed you.

Be aware of the environment - pay attention to the space where you are eating, the table, the decor, light, sounds. You will never again wish to inhale your meal in front of the TV or hidden in the pantry.

Make a new rule - eat only when you are at peace, in a good mood, and present in the moment. Before you take something to eat, take some time to set yourself, and contemplate for a few moments. Your wish for food may disappear, and you find out there's something else you need. You'll become aware of your thoughts and emotions that made you think you are hungry in the first place. If you still want to eat, it's ok, and you will be in the right mood for food, present, conscious, and calm.

## Love yourself

You have probably heard this many times. And maybe you think it's ridiculous - of course I love myself, everybody loves themselves. But, that's not quite the truth. Actually, you would be surprised if you realized how little love most people have for themselves. We are generally better with others, often putting their needs before ours, we are more kind, empathetic, and loving with others than with the most important person in our lives - ourselves. How is this possible? We learned it. As a baby, you adored yourself. Babies know how precious, loved, and miraculous they are. A baby thinks he or she is the center of the universe, and he or she requires their needs to be met. They don't care if someone doesn't like their screaming. They are the most important thing in the world, and they insist on getting what they need. But later, we learn (sometimes it's correct, sometimes wrong) that we are not the center of the universe, that our needs are not so important, that we are not worthy, not so loved, not acceptable, and so on. Some of that is necessary for us to learn if we want to become a part of society. Some of those beliefs are far from the truth, but they seem entirely true for us when we are three. All those things we learn and start to believe about ourselves make us love ourselves less. We live with a feeling of inadequacy, worthlessness, insecurity, shyness, and a lack of love. That makes us put many mental barriers in our way, and we struggle all the time. We believe we are solving problems all the time, while we are actually making them. What we need is to learn again how worthy and precious we are. We need to love ourselves and our uniqueness again. How can we do that?

First, do a lot of introspection and dig up everything you believe about yourself. All the embarrassing things, all you hate about yourself, all you need to forgive yourself. Don't be surprised if it is a long list.

Then forgive yourself. Forgive yourself for every mistake and failure, for all your weaknesses and flaws.

Sit still, relax, and breathe. Imagine another you is coming. Talk to the other you. Tell her or him that you are forgiving. Imagine you two are hugging, bathed in healing, white light. Then let your old self go back to the past.

If you don't feel ready to forgive, don't worry. Repeat an affirmation, "I'm ready to forgive myself," until you really feel that it becomes true.

For each negative belief you have about yourself, create an affirmation to replace it. For example, instead of, "I'm ugly; I'm stupid; I never do things right; I'm worthless; No'one could ever love me," try, "now I recognize how wonderful I am. I am gorgeous. I'm smart, intelligent, wise, and divinely guided. Things are always happening for my highest good. I'm worth love. Now I know how worthy I am. I love, and I'm loved. I deserve love. I deserve to be happy. I give and receive love." Repeat affirmations in front of the mirror. That way, your subconscious will easier accept them as the truth because you are hearing them from a real person, with the eye contact, the same way you heard things you started believing as a child.

Meditation will also help you go a long way in building self-love, self-esteem, and confidence. In meditation, you may discover your limiting beliefs, old patterns, and blocks you have to work on.

Once you learn to love yourself, your whole life will change. You will make different choices that lead to your good, do different things that make you happy, and find new ways to fill your life with joy. You will become your best friend and your most significant support. Once you change your inner talk from your worst enemy into a loving friend, you'll unlock your hidden potential.

## Express yourself

Like accumulated experiences that may manifest as extra weight, our unexpressed feelings and unrealized ideas can get the same results.

What's your way of expressing yourself? Do you do art? Painting, drawing, dancing, playing an instrument, writing? If you like something, do you make time for it? If you don't do that, consider starting. Sign up for a drawing course or dance class. It's never too late to start acting or singing. Find your passion, something that makes time stand still. If you have no idea what makes you happy, recall what you loved to do as a child. Did you like to play roles, to paint, to make up stories, or to read? Perhaps that activity would make the adult you happy. Any artistic activity will allow you to express yourself. It may sound strange, but it can help you lose weight or maintain your ideal weight.

Besides expressing yourself, joyful artistic activities have proven effects on finding inner peace. That has an extra indirect impact on your weight loss.

"Lose your weight writing, dance your weight down, sing out your weight" - could you imagine a better way to lose some extra pounds?

## Break boredom

Boredom is a trivial, but significant, reason for snacking and overeating. If your life is dull, you feel stuck, not excited at all, lack enthusiasm, it's time to make some changes.

Boredom usually comes in the package with a lack of sense and purpose. Try to find your passion and your purpose. If you do something meaningful that you enjoy and believe you are making a difference in the world, you will hardly ever be bored.

But everybody happens to have a dull day, to get exhausted by repeating the same routine over and over again. Step out from your usual routine and do something different. Ride a bike, feed birds, talk to a colleague you have never chatted to before, or take your kids to the zoo, whatever you don't repeat every day.

There are many different things you can do and activities you can take to overcome boredom, whether it's momentary or constant.

Here is a list of ideas of what you could do instead of snacking:
- go out for a walk
- sing your favorite song
- call a friend
- do 20 squats
- do 5 minutes of exercise
- drink a glass of water
- water a flower
- play with kids or pets
- read 10 pages of a book
- draw something
- turn on music and dance
- do some quick tidying or dusting
- meditate
- take a shower
- do a plank
- do some yoga
- listen to a podcast
- write your journey of gratitude.

These are just some ideas. Be creative, try out different things, and see what's working for you. The point is to turn your attention to something else instead of food.

## Diet from negativity and develop a positive mindset

Cutting out negative thoughts and toxic feelings will do more for your health, the weight included, than cutting out calories. While a lower-calorie intake can work miracles for weight loss, the lower consumption of negativity is crucial for maintaining your healthy weight.

So, commit yourself to inner work. Do introspection and question your thoughts and feelings. Change negative beliefs into positive ones that will serve you. Do everything you need to reach a good mood and positive vibe - meditate, write a journal of gratitude, visualize your desired scenario. Focus on the good side of everything and try to find the best in everyone and every situation. Believe in a higher, divine power, whatever it means for you. Believing that you are divinely protected and guided for the highest good and greatest joy will bring you more peace than you could imagine.

Find power hidden in yourself - the power of life, your willpower, and the power of love. Knowing the power is within you makes all the fears smaller, and brings the peace, too.

Avoid negative people, negative news, and all the negativity you can, and feed your mind with a lot of positive and loving thoughts. This will heal your soul, and, as the change must begin from the inside, your body will experience the change, too.

All those techniques we were talking about will help you develop a positive mindset. You are not determined to think a certain way. You can learn and practice being an optimist, and a happy person. You can learn how to find inner peace. Like every muscle in our body, our mind needs to be trained to stay in good shape. Positive thinking requires a lot of inner work and daily practice. But it quickly pays off - your mind will change, and your whole life becomes different. Spiritual and mindful awaking is the best thing you can do for yourself, including not just your soul and the mind, but also your body, because it's a mirror reflection of what is in the inside.

## Conclusion

While the traditional approach to weight loss focuses only on the body, calories in versus calories out, like it's a separated mechanism, in this book, we suggest a different, unconventional approach - a holistic one. You shouldn't take your body as if it's an isolated device, unconnected with your mind and the soul. It's a part of a bigger picture, and you should think about it that way. Being overweight is a symptom of deeper issues. So, if you want to become and stay fit forever, you shouldn't stay at the surface. You should begin from the inside.

What we suggest as a universal cure for many problems, including weight, is finding inner peace. Once you become happy, calm, mindful, balanced and satisfied, the healthy lifestyle and healthy weight will follow, as a natural consequence of your correct mindset.

Printed in Great Britain
by Amazon

53753852R00028